UNKINKED

By

Cathy Brown

TABLE OF CONTENTS

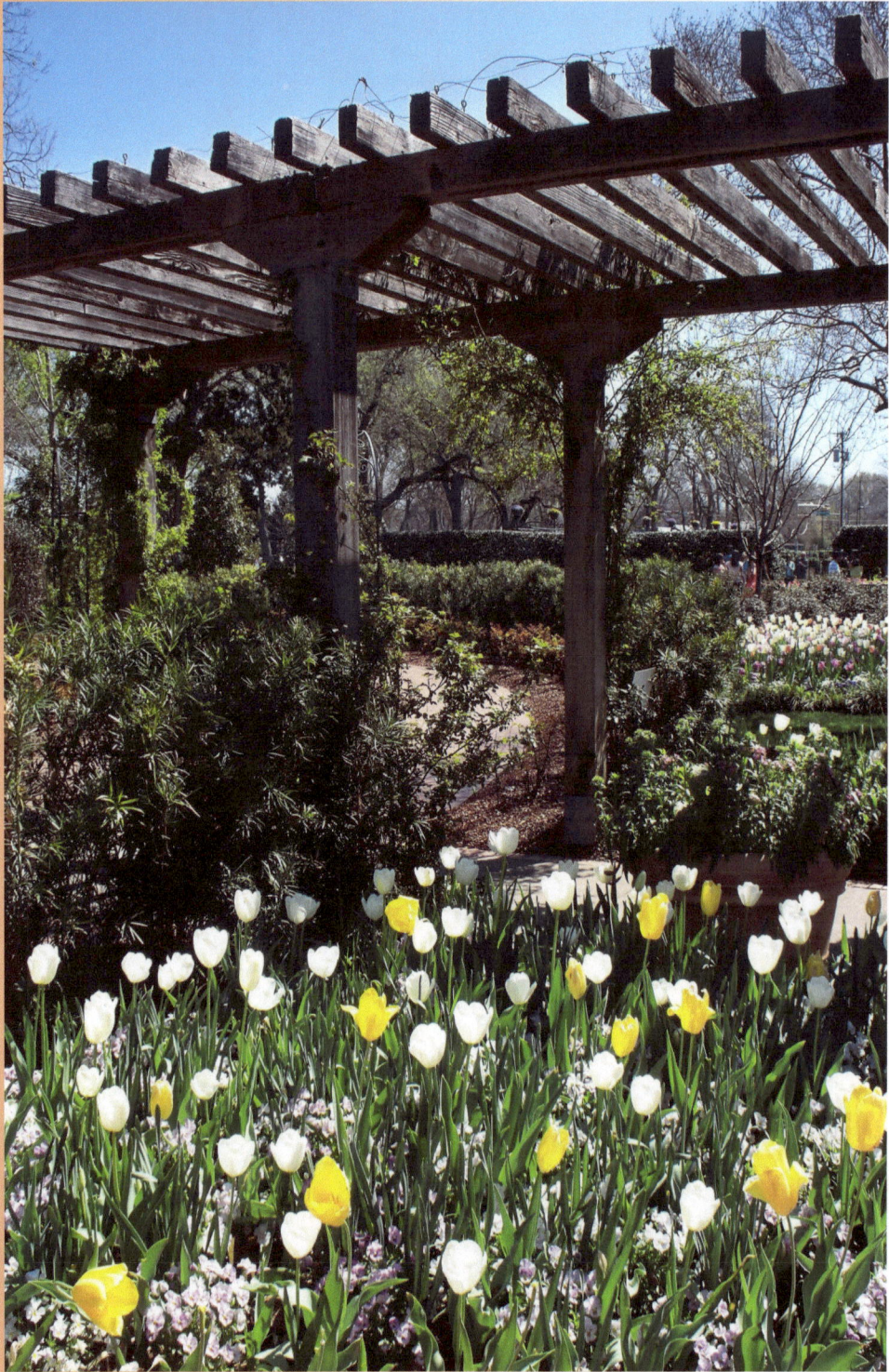

Preface

You deserve to know something about the author! My name is Cathy Brown. First, of all I am a daughter, a sister, a wife, a mother, and a grandparent. I have had the challenge of raising a blended family. And for 30 years, like many of you, I have tried to juggle a demanding career, as well.

My story begins like this---Due to the interruptions of marriage and childbirth, my college education was not actually accomplished until my late twenties. So I started out my career at the age of 28 with a husband and 3 children under the age of 7 to keep me busy.   My career was so exciting that I could hardly believe that I was finally living my dream and getting paid for it, too! For years, I stayed home with the kids during the week and worked every weekend. Even though my husband also worked hard, there was NEVER a day off and no time/money for vacations. Sure, I felt fulfilled and useful in my life, but it WAS a chaotic existence.   Oh well... when you are young, you can do almost anything-thank goodness! ... NOW, LET'S FAST-FORWARD A FEW YEARS...By my late-thirties, I found myself to be a single mother, raising 4 children from the ages of 16 to 8 years old. Now I was forced to work full-time outside the home. If life had been chaotic before, it was hugely magnified now. There were many days that I just rolled my eyes back, thinking that the world was revolving too fast to jump off, even for just a short rest. And no end was in sight! As time went on, I was offered a position in which I would be a stress management coach for my co-workers, in addition to my usual duties, of course. So, I set out to become more knowledgeable about that topic. And as I learned, I shared with my fellow employees.

My purpose for this workbook is to help you learn ways to benefit from **current** information about stress management, using the well-known Mayo Clinic as resource material at http://www.mayoclinic.org/healthy-living/stress-management/basics/stress-basics/hlv-20049495. (Just for your information, this UNKINKED Workbook has no association with Mayo Clinic or any affiliated Mayo entity.)   I have designed practical worksheets to help you incorporate healthy concepts of daily living into your lifestyle. If you just read the information, you will be more knowledgeable, but information that is not used is basically worthless.   So, I would like to encourage you to PRACTISE what you learn. And now it is time to get started!

UNKINKED-   Introduction

WELCOME TO <u>UNKINKED</u>!

I think it would be fair to say that one of the most overwhelming challenges that our society today faces is the taming of a monster called "STRESS". Most of us are on a merry-go-round that is headed in a circle, going nowhere, and moving so fast that there is just no way to get off. So, how does that look?

- Employers advertise for workers who are ready to work in a "fast-paced environment".

- Being able to multi-task is a much sought after quality trait in an employee.

- There seems to be rampant discontent in the workplace, with employees feeling increasing levels of pressure to perform better and faster.

- So many of us are stressed because of long work hours or because we don't feel like a part of something really worthwhile, past just earning an income.

- Some of us yearn to be able to use our gifts and abilities, but, instead, we feel stifled by our bosses, who tend to micro-manage away our creativity.

- And then, when we finally do get home after a long day's work, we start to multi-task all over again. Even then, there is not enough time to do more than the bare essentials at home.

- Our marriages are suffering and our children are neglected.

- Maintaining any kind of friendships is barely possible, simply because we have no energy left.

STRESS IS PERSONAL!

List some ways stress affects YOU personally…

1.

2.

3.

4.

5.

Then list the three things/areas that **cause** most of your own stress symptoms...

1.

2.

3.

(It is important to customize this workbook to meet your own personal needs by FOCUSING on the areas that you have listed just now.)

Stress Levels Are Influenced By:

How we conduct our lives

How we think about things

How we nurture ourselves

Some Common Effects of Stress

Body:

Muscle tension   Headache   Chest pain

Stomach upset   Fatigue

Mood:

Irritability   Restlessness   Anxiety

Depression   Inability to focus

Behavior:

Overeating   Tobacco use   Angry outbursts

Alcohol abuse   Social withdrawal

NATURE IS A NATURAL STRESS REDUCER

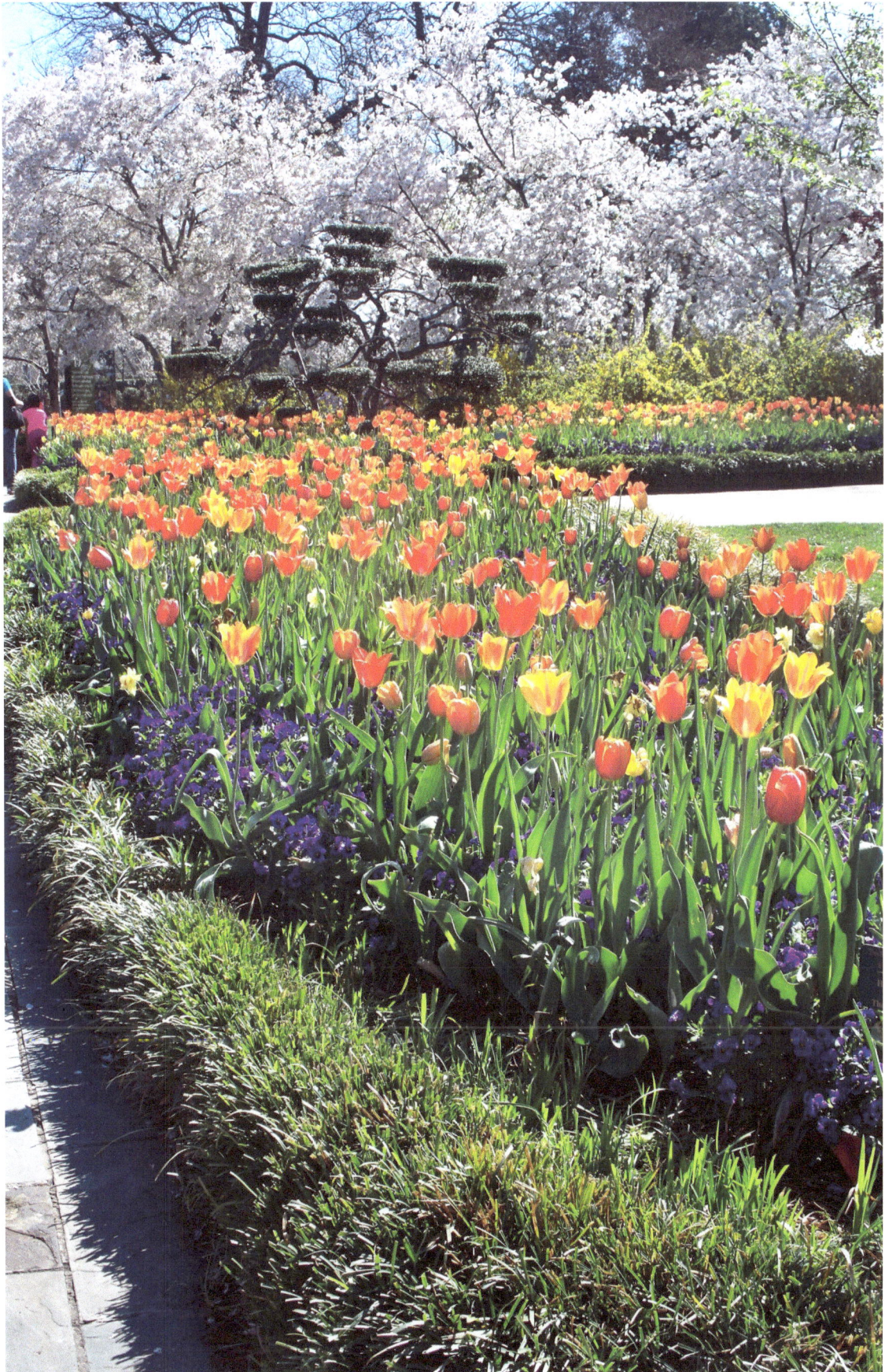

Chapter One

THE GRATITUDE FACTOR

EVERY DAY IS A GIFT! How much thought do we really give to the gifts in our lives? Why not take a few moments each day to let those gifts sink in… to our minds/hearts? Forming a habit like this one can go a <u>long</u> way toward decreasing our stress levels.

Whenever we have our "oasis" times during the day-whether it is in the morning, or during breaks throughout the day or in the evenings-this is a good time to purposely think about the good things in our lives.

One day, I met a businessman in a really high-stress field who had an interesting way to squeeze in his little "oasis" during the work day. During a conversation, he began to tell me how much he loved to take photos of his vacations. He said that he loads them into his computer at work and looks at them there. Immediately, I realized that this must be the way he decompresses at work. Obviously, he uses "visualization" to rest his mind for a few minutes at whatever times he has available.

Whether he realized it or not, this man was practicing stress management, by reliving the good parts of his life---the things he is thankful for. He had discovered a way to reinforce the beauty in his life over and over in a way that would not only give him pleasure, but would also calm and refresh him on a frequent basis.

Have you noticed that you feel more relaxed, less anxious, and more contented during the moments you're thinking about the good things in your life?

After you've made a list of things you are thankful for, then what? Well, we asserted that thinking grateful/thankful thoughts makes us feel better---as long as we are thinking about them. But how can we make those feelings last longer?

Consider that whatever we are thankful for, can serve as an invitation to give back in some way.

GRATITUDE IS POWERFUL!

Make a list of 6 specific things that you are grateful for…

1.

2.

3.

4.

5.

6.

Make a list of 6 specific things that you can <u>do</u> with those thankful thoughts...

1.

2.

3.

4.

5.

6.

Pick one of those specific things to do each week. Chances are that you will begin to feel MORE POWERFUL and LESS STRESSED yourself!

Chapter Two

THE SOLITUDE FACTOR

I once read about a real woman who lived a number of years ago, who had ten children. For years, the best she could do to get some solitude was to raise her apron up over her head to cover her face so that she could chill out for a moment. Have you ever felt that desperate? Well, that reminds me of the mother whose child took her time to start talking, but eventually, she chattered non-stop all day long while following her mother around the house. Apparently, the little girl put words to every single thought that came into her mind. The frazzled mother hated to put a stop to it, not wanting her child to feel unimportant, so she listened until it felt like her ears were reamed out-no solitude here!

Have you ever thought about the impact of noise in your life? There was a time when my husband and I were considering the purchase of an gasoline generator for emergencies and for our camping trips. One of the factors we researched concerned how loud the generator would be. We found that some of them registered at decibels that are supposedly hazardous to your health, leading to hearing loss. Not only that, we were told that too much noise can increase blood pressure, as well as increase the risk of tinnitus (ringing in the ears) and other problems like a stroke or a heart attack. Now it would take further research to verify all of these statements, but I am sure we all have some understanding of the ill effects of noise. How many of you have noticed feeling tense, irritable, or even aggressive when being exposed to noise that is too loud, too frequent, or too continuous? How many of you have had trouble relaxing or sleeping or just concentrating in the presence of too much noise? So, would you say that noise can be disruptive in your life?

When was the last time you were completely and blissfully ALONE for a few minutes at some place besides the restroom?

Have you forgotten what the sound of silence is like? Are you comfortable alone with your own thoughts?

Does the thought of spending a large segment of time without human company make you feel uneasy?

Please allow me to quote a description of solitude that I wrote in a previous work. It goes like this:

"I have found a way to actually look forward to my busy days. Instead of jumping out of bed at the last minute, I have learned to set the alarm for one hour earlier than it takes me to get ready for the day. (Of course, it helps to go to bed an hour earlier, provided there is nothing good to watch on television. Ha!). I stumble into the kitchen to begin my soothing morning ritual of putting coffee on to brew; somehow, I enjoy this mindless task, probably because it helps me ease into the day. Next, comes my predictable bowl of cereal and milk; and for a special treat, I sometimes add fresh fruit. By this time, the aroma of coffee is permeating the kitchen. So, I pour a cup, add some cream, and take it to the couch where I sit down and slowly savor my exotic liquid dessert! In the quiet of the morning, I just sit there, sipping and relaxing, thinking about nothing except the moment. Soon I become more aware of my surroundings and find myself marveling about things normally taken for granted; I hear the birds chirping outside, the clock chiming on the hour, and my husband beginning his own morning routine in the shower. Shortly thereafter, he joins me to share a second cup of coffee TOGETHER before the concerns of the day demand our attention. What a blissful way to start each new day!"

Stress is inevitable and it takes a terrible toll on our mood, body, and behavior. But there is so much that we can do to <u>negate</u> those destructive effects. We can nurture ourselves back to better health and well-being. And it can begin with **solitude**.

WHAT WOULD SOLITUDE LOOK LIKE IN YOUR LIFE?

List some ways that you can make a little time each day for periods of solitude:

1.

2.

3.

As you make your list:

Try to be creative. Don't expect to find a perfect scenario. Be willing to schedule more than one short "oasis" throughout the day when a single long one is not practical. Enlist other people to help you fit this time into your life.

WATER HAS A CALMING EFFECT

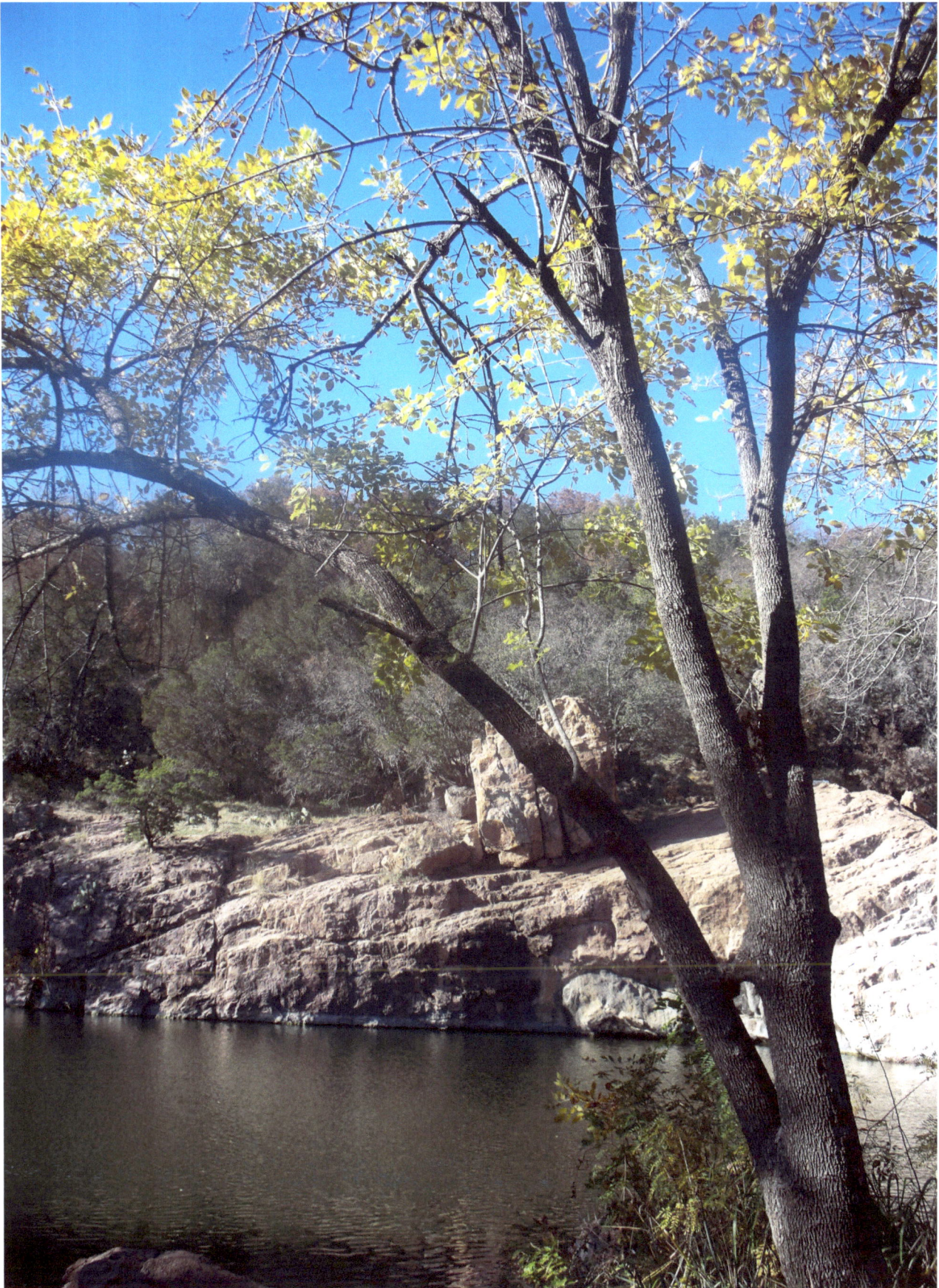

Chapter Three

THE SABOTAGE FACTOR

We can set ourselves up for stress by:

Procrastination

Negative self-talk

Disorganization

Misaligned priorities

Over-scheduling

Ineffective communication

Co-dependence

A sedentary lifestyle

Ingratitude

Limited "down time"

Excessive caffeine

Multi-tasking

Poor listening skills

ARE YOU YOUR OWN WORST ENEMY?

We Sabotage Ourselves by How We Self-Nurture:

1. Sedentary lifestyle
2.
3.
4.

We Sabotage Ourselves by How We Think:

1. Negative self-talk
2.
3.

We Sabotage Ourselves by How We Conduct Our Lives:

1. Procrastination
2.
3.
4.
5.

Using the previous page, please fill in these blanks.

Chapter Four

THE PURPOSE FACTOR

Is there something more to life?

Maybe you have longed to embrace a greater purpose than just pursuing your own happiness or fame or fortune.

Would you feel more fulfilled if you were building a meaningful legacy to pass on to others?

Medical science suggests that people who have a clear focus that is BEYOND themselves, tend to weather stress better.

But HOW do you find YOUR special purpose in life?

My Story:

While I was job hunting several years ago, a family member told me about a job opportunity at the company where he worked. It was something I had <u>never</u>, in my wildest dreams, contemplated; but out of respect for him, I began the interview process. As I sat through one session after another, I began to see how my past experiences and interests made me uniquely qualified to fill that position. It was as if I had been created specifically for this particular job! Realizing that completely changed my perspective, allowing me the courage to venture into uncharted territory. I would be a part of a long needed service to others that had never been pursued in the industry before. Needless to say, it became one of the most satisfying jobs of my whole career!

Light Bulb Moment:

Consider that you already have a hint as to what YOUR unique purpose in life might be. In your search for purpose, start with what you already have.

START WITH WHAT YOU ALREADY HAVE

Use this space to write out your answers:

1. List your interests.   What topics energize you?

2. Discuss your strengths. What do you feel confident in?

3. Consider your unique knowledge.   Do you have information that few people are privy to?

4. Make use of your present skills.   What are they?

5. Ask yourself what new things you would like to learn. Write them down here.

6. Enlist your friends and family. What do **they** think you have to offer?

THE ANIMAL CONNECTION IS NURTURING

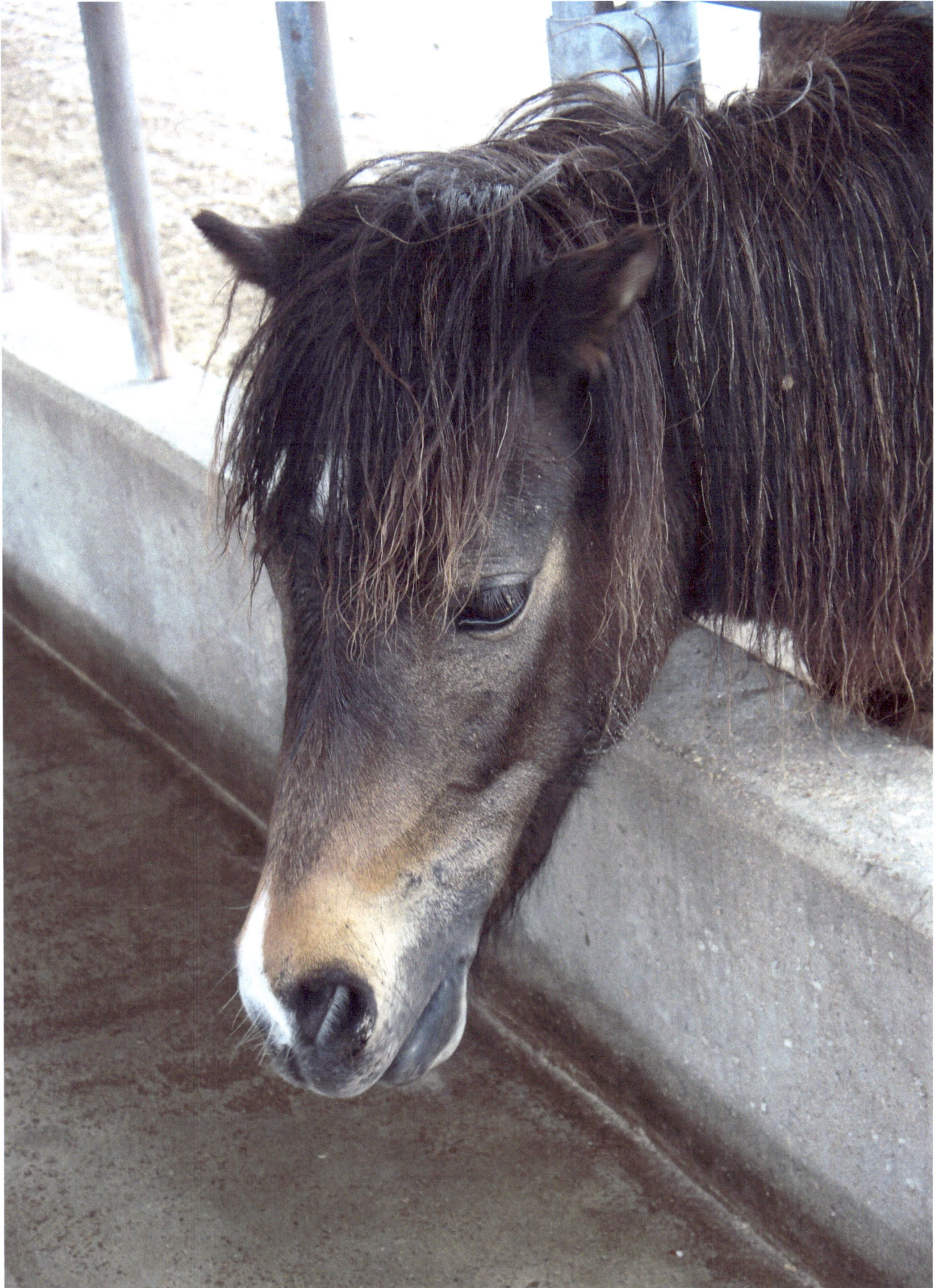

Chapter Five

THE TIME FACTOR

MISALIGNED PRIORITIES
PROCRASTINATION
OVER-SCHEDULING
DISORGANIZATION
MULTI-TASKING
DISTRACTIONS

Does this list speak to your own daily life?

All of the traits above contribute to poor use of the time allotted for each 24 hour day. Fortunately, all of them will respond to one thing....FOCUS!

Focus on your top priorities…First, concentrate on the three things that are most important in the long run. Don't allow urgent tasks to take up so much time that the top priorities are neglected.

Focus on action…Procrastination is tempting when faced with a large project, so break it up into smaller tasks until the project is completed.

Focus on a realistic schedule…Be fair to yourself and your clients by giving yourself more time than you expect to need. If you finish early, it gives your clients more confidence in you.

Focus on orderliness…Disorganization wastes precious time!   Taking a few minutes to get organized in the beginning tends to make the project or task progress more smoothly and faster.

Focus on one thing at a time...When you give your undivided attention to whatever you are working on, distractions are less likely and then the quality of your work tends to go up.

TIME IS A PRECIOUS RESOURCE!

1. What are YOUR top three priorities?

2. How can you break up that large project that you are dreading into smaller and more manageable segments?

3. Imagine your client's reaction when you finished their project earlier than you promised. How do you think that would affect your future business?

4. Where are the areas in your work day that could benefit from a more organized approach?

5. If you focused on one project at a time, how would it make your day look different?

Would you be willing to try it for a period of time, just to see how it could decrease your stress, contribute to your satisfaction with life, and increase your productivity in the long run? Where will you start?

Chapter Six

THE EXERCISE FACTOR

Stress is an unfortunate part of living; however, it is very responsive to the way we react to it. It can cause a variety of symptoms like tight shoulder muscles, headaches, depression, and even weight gain. One of my favorite ways to deal with it is … exercise.

Question:

How does exercise help with stress?

Answer:

It helps us react in a more constructive way.

****

Question:

But HOW does it help us deal more effectively with stress?

Answer:

1. It helps our bodies to release physical tension. Have you ever noticed that taking a brisk walk or doing some other aerobic activity makes your muscles feel less tense?

2. It redirects our thoughts/emotions to something physical. That alone, can be quite therapeutic. Getting "outside of our heads" can be just the kind of break that we need to tackle stressors with fresh insights and renewed vigor.

EXERCISE WORKS MAGIC!

When people have sedentary jobs, they may be at a higher risk for stress symptoms than those who are more active. Frequent and regular exercise can go a long way toward protecting us from the stresses of everyday living. One of the best ways to make a habit of exercise is to find a variety of activities that are enjoyable.   Then swap them out to keep it interesting. So what are YOUR favorite types of exercise?

1.

2.

3.

4.

What are some ways that you can incorporate more exercise into your lifestyle?

1.

2.

3.

4.

WALKING RELIEVES MUSCLE TENSION

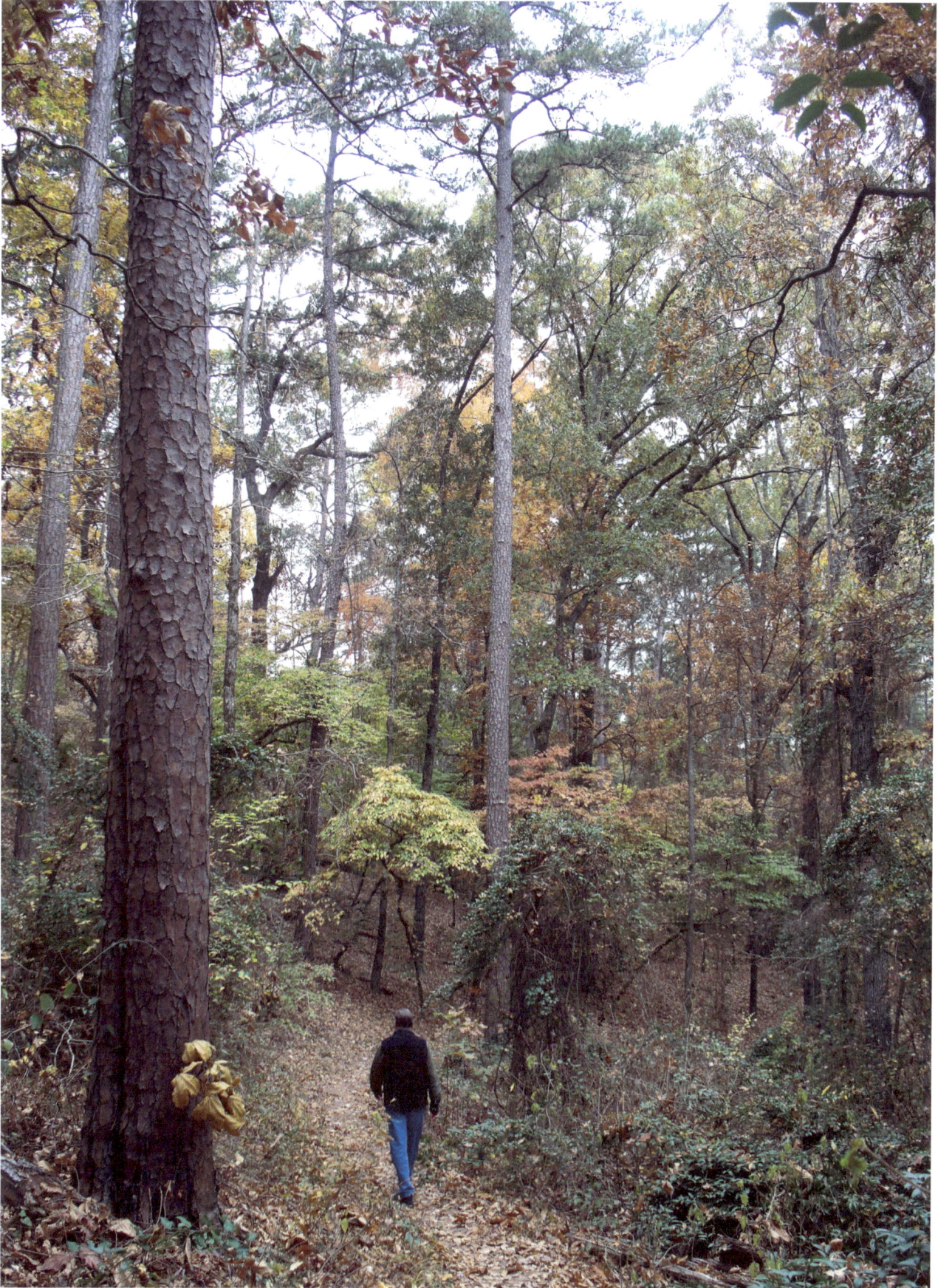

Chapter Seven

THE MINDFULNESS FACTOR

What IS Mindfulness?

It is giving full attention to what you are experiencing every moment.

How does that translate?

- While you are driving….think about being a safe driver instead of texting or talking on the cell phone or instead of daydreaming about your next vacation.

- As you make dinner...think about preparing an attractive, nutritious meal instead of planning your activities for the next day.

- When you take the dog out to do his business….spend a full 30 minutes to notice nature all around you instead of rushing back inside.

- During the process of completing a task...limit interruptions instead of multi-tasking.

These are just a few of the ways that we often dilute the pleasure of the moment. What a shame to waste one of the most valuable aspects of life….the gift of the present   The past is gone and the future is not promised. But we do have the NOW. So, why not fully enjoy it?

Focusing on the present is also a good way to decrease stress, because it temporarily gives us a break from thoughts of the past (like regret, etc.) and thoughts of the future (like worry, etc.). In other words, it allows us to take a rest. It is not an excuse to ignore things that we need to think through, but it does help us to replenish ourselves, so that we can take better ownership of those things at a time that we have set aside to brainstorm or to ponder on them. Focusing on the present can help us to live life with more satisfaction, with more intent, and with more success!

Look at Each Moment as a Treasure!

LIVING IN THE MOMENT

Your assignment for this week is to PRACTISE thinking about only what you are experiencing during the time you are taking your bath or shower. Do this every day for the next week. Instead of thinking about what you have to do during the day, etc., just keep bringing your thoughts back to the experience of your bath time; you may be surprised at how little time you spend actually thinking about this daily routine. And you may find it challenging to stay focused on it; but when you do, it can be enlightening to realize how much you have been taking for granted. So try this experiment—walk into the bathroom as if you were seeing if for the first time (just like you do when you notice the details of your accommodations while on vacation). Use each of your five senses (sight, hearing, smell, taste, touch). Take a few minutes each day to write down something that you did not notice before.

You may use the items listed below to help you concentrate on the experience:

- What does the bathroom <u>look</u> like? (Notice colors, textures, shapes, lighting, etc.)

- What flavors can you <u>taste</u>? (Toothpaste, mouth wash, dental floss, etc.)

- What sensations do you <u>feel</u> on your skin? (Bubbles, warmth, pulling, stinging, etc.)

- What <u>smells</u> do you encounter? (Soap, shampoo, shaving cream, skin lotion, cosmetics, etc.)

CONCLUSION

Stress management is one of the most important skills that any person can learn. It affects, not only our physical health, but also our mental well-being. Furthermore, it tends to add both length and quality to our lives.

Spanning all aspects of our every moment, it is a never-ending quest to keep our lives balanced . But when we continue to keep focusing on how to best deal with our stress, we can't help but enjoy life more fully. Fortunately, it does not take perfection to make a significant improvement!

As parents and grandparents, we are in a position to demonstrate healthy living skills by our own example. While we spend fortunes on a college education that can provide our adult children with a career, how much time and money do we expend teaching them how to live their lives SUCCESSFULLY in other areas? Most of us really try hard, but we just don't have the knowledge or experience to pass on to them.

No matter what the ages of our children—-whether a toddler or a forty-year-old executive, it is never too early or too late to make a difference. By learning to manage stress better ourselves, we have made the first step toward enriching the lives of our family members. Congratulations to us all!

APPENDIX

OTHER WORKS BY CATHY BROWN

This author presents a variety of stress management tools, hoping to enhance the everyday life of her readers. They include works for adults (self-help), for children (adventure/fiction), and for the family (a choice of calendar topics designed to interest all ages and sexes). Liberal use of colorful photographs and designs have been utilized for your reading pleasure. Her latest literary and photographic publications are available for a free preview at lulu.com. And watch for her books on the Amazon and Barnes & Noble websites as well.

BOOKS

Just Thinking

The gift of life...what is it all about? Have you ever wondered why you were born? Do you feel compelled to find answers to your questions about your origin and purpose? Take a little time each day to learn how to nurture your own spirituality, while you marvel over 20-plus amazing, beautiful, and inspiring photographs.

Andy's Camping Adventure

Come along with six-year-old Andy on his first camping trip! Feel his excitement as a scavenger hunt leads him to buried treasure. And use the clues to figure out what was causing the mysterious reappearing animal tracks. It was an experience that changed his family life forever...for the better!

A Calendar of Jewels

It is amazing what the scribbles on your old calendars can reveal! They are almost like reading your own personal diary. When I looked through some of my own old calendars, suddenly I saw the bigger picture of my life in a way that gave me more hope. And hope is a great stress reducer, because it gives birth to patience and resilience. So, why not leaf through some of your own old calendars to see what jewels YOU can discover?

REFERENCES—MAYO CLINIC

Basics---http://www.mayoclinic.org/healthy-living/stress-management/basics/stress-basics/hlv-20049495 (2014)

Health---http://www.mayoclinic.org/healthy-living/stress-management/in-depth/stress/art-20046037 (2013)

Adult health---http://www.mayoclinic.org/healthy-living/adult-health/basics/staying-healthy/hlv-20049421 (2014)

Sources of stress---http://www.mayoclinic.org/healthy-living/stress-management/in-depth/stress-management/art-20044151 (2013)

Sabotage---http://www.mayoclinic.org/healthy-living/stress-management/in-depth/health-tip/art-20048653 (2013)

Sabotage/Saying No---http://www.mayoclinic.org/healthy-living/stress-management/in-depth/stress-relief/art-20044494 (2013)

Sabotage/Preventing setbacks---http://www.mayoclinic.org/healthy-living/stress-management/in-depth/stress-management/art-20044489 (2013)

Solitude/Spirituality---http://www.mayoclinic.org/healthy-living/stress-management/in-depth/stress-relief/art-20044464?pg=2 (2013)

Focus---http://www.mayoclinic.org/healthy-living/adult-health/expert-answers/how-to-focus/faq-20058383 (2012)

www.ingramcontent.com/pod-product-compliance
Lightning Source LLC
Chambersburg PA
CBHW042007080426
42733CB00003B/36